HCG Diet

Carl Preston

DISCLAIMER

This book details the author's personal experiences with and opinions about right-brained learning. The author is not licensed as an educational consultant, teacher, psychologist, or psychiatrist.

The author and publisher are providing this book and its contents on an "as is" basis and make no representations or warranties of any kind with respect to this book or its contents. The author and publisher disclaim all such representations and warranties, including for example warranties of merchantability and educational or medical advice for a particular purpose. In addition, the author and publisher do not represent or warrant that the information accessible via this book is accurate, complete or current.

The statements made about products and services have not been evaluated by the U.S. government. Please consult with your own legal or accounting professional regarding the suggestions and recommendations made in this book.

Except as specifically stated in this book, neither the author or publisher, nor any authors, contributors, or other representatives will be liable for damages arising out of or in connection with the use of this book. This is a comprehensive limitation of liability that applies to all damages of any kind, including (without limitation) compensatory; direct, indirect or consequential damages; loss of data, income or profit; loss of or damage to property and claims of third parties.

You understand that this book is not intended as a substitute for consultation with a licensed medical, educational, legal or accounting professional. Before you begin any change in your lifestyle in any way, you will consult a licensed professional to ensure that you are doing what's best for your situation.

This book provides content related to educational, medical, and psychological topics. As such, use of this book implies your acceptance of this disclaimer.

Contents

The Benefits of the HCG Diet

So you have decided to take on the HCG diet and to transform your life forever. Here are the benefits you will reap from following the HCG Diet to the letter. You will:

- Achieve an extremely fast weight loss (5 lbs/week average!
- You will not only lose pounds, but those inches making you feel tight in your cloths will be gone
- You will go through a very low calorie diet having minor or no hunger at all, thanks to HCG.
- You will not need to exercise.
- You will be able to tackle stubborn fat deposits. They will be gone forever!
- You will look great: Slimmer, healthier and more confident than ever.
- Your energy levels will rocket up, and you will be able to be much more physical in y our daily life.
- You will discover and maintain healthier and better habits.
- You will save money on gym fees, expensive dieting food and homeopathy visits.

Frequently Asked Questions

What does HCG mean?

Human Chorionic Gonadotropin (HCG) is a hormone that's produce in pregnant women by the placenta and by the hypothalamus in order to regulate metabolic rates within a person's system. HCG derivatives are commonly used in treating fertility issues by assisting in getting women pregnant. For this diet, another derivative of this hormone is created to aid in natural weight loss for those needing to reduce their body mass.

By using this hormone to regulate metabolic rates, a person can see dramatic results in a relatively short time period. In order to complete this diet, blood tests are usually required by a physician to assess a person's tolerance towards the injections of this hormone.

Once a person is cleared by a physician, they are free to work towards this diet's main objectives: to lose weight and to lower or eliminate the risks associated with overweight individuals.

How does HCG affect the body so that you lose weight?

HCG works on regulating a person's metabolic rate by breaking down fats from the adipose tissue of a person's body. Adipose tissue is the area that's responsible for all the unsightly weight gain that can be seen on a person.

By breaking down the fats stored here instead of lean muscle (some other diets break down this as well), a person can see weight loss results without the added worry that their stored protein levels are in jeopardy, only their stored fat levels.

As it breaks down these stored fats, the hormone is also releasing these fats back into the bloodstream so that they are burned off throughout the day's activities. Since HCG only focuses on stored fats, an individual doesn't have to worry about losing other important nutrients or their muscle mass while working through this diet.

Who can use this diet? Are there any exclusions?

This diet can be utilized by both men and women though a visit to a physician is recommended before starting HCG injections or other HCG protocols.

When consulting a physician, one should go over their weight along with their options in order to ensure this diet is a viable choice for that person.

However, pregnant and/or nursing women won't be able to participate due to their current conditions though they are eligible once they conclude their pregnancy and/or nursing phases.

What are the risks and side effects of this diet?

As with all diets, there are pros and cons to each, and the same can be said for the HCG diet. Starting with the pros of this diet, they include achieving the diet's primary goal in losing the extra weight, lowering the health risks of obesity, and stabling of blood sugar, along with increased metabolism and energy.

Losing the weight and lowering health risks are the objectives that most strive to achieve with this diet since they are close to living through the nightmarish risks of being obese, such as high blood pressure and even diabetes.

As for the cons of HCG injections, these can include injection site redness and/or swelling and headaches, which are mainly attributed to the meal plan for this diet and the low calorie intake that this diet requires to be successful.

There is also a chance for Ovarian Hyper stimulation Syndrome (OHSS), but this far more likely when HCG is instrumental in fertility procedures because of the high doses needed. The diet uses considerably lower dosages for those participating.

When on this diet protocol, it's important to discuss any drugs that are being taken so as to evaluate their possible interactions with the HCG hormone.

The cons of ingestible HCG sublingual serums include headaches, constipation, and indigestion. Some of the same cons are also found in the diet's menu plan with the inclusion of dizziness, muscle cramps, and even a rash.

Your HCG Treatment Options

HCG Injections	HCG Sublingual Drops	HCG Pellets/Pills	HCG Sprays
1- 3 Pounds Daily Weight loss	1- 3 Pounds Daily Weight loss	Results not verifiable yet	Results not verifiable yet
Effective	Effective	Less effective than drops and injections	Less effective than drops injections and pellets
Injected through needle. People with needle phobia should strictly avoid this form.	Under the tongue	Swallowed with water.	Sprayed under tongue.
They have expiry date. Low shelf life	No expiry date. Great shelf life	They have expiry date. Medium shelf life	They have expiry date. Low shelf life
Itchiness, Infections and swelling from injections.	Homeopathic HCG drops are prepared after a rigorous dilution process. Hence they are completely safe.	Can cause starvation.	Can cause fatigue.
Muscle cramps, lumps and pain. Dizziness, nausea and vomiting.	No cramps and pain. No side-effects during HCG diet	Mild Headache and fatigue	Dizziness, nausea and vomiting. Mild headache

The HCG Dosage

There are standard doses depending on what intake method for the hormone you use:

- .125-175 dose of hCG
- 125iu-175 2x per day if sublingual
- 6 drops 3x per day if homeopathic

However this can be varying. You mays start with a different dosage, or even move it up or down during the low calorie process (phase2). Men usually cant ber around 0.025-0.050 higher than women.

You can find your sweet spot by checking how and when you feel hungry during the 500 calorie intake process.

Finding the right dosage

- If you were to start at 125iu and you felt very hungry, that would be a pretty easy fix as raising the dose, since 125iu is the lowest used.
- Starting with 150iu HCG, you may need an increase or decrease. If you are feeling hungry especially towards the end of the day, that means your dose of the hormone is too low and you need to increase it. If it happens early in the day it means you need to lower it.
- If you were started on a lower dose in the range of doses that people in general feel better with, between 125 iu-175iu but are feeling hunger, I would start out with minor adjustments of 25-50ius. A too high or too low does will make you feel starving.
- A more reliable possibly quicker way to know what dose change to make, once the hormone has been in your system already for at least a week, Is to skip a dose entirely one day. That will make it pretty clear- if your hunger is much better on the day you skip a dose, you need less HCG.

The HCG Diet Phases

Phase 1 or Loading Phase

While taking your HCG dose, you eat as high fat as possible, reaching even to the point of nausea, for 2-3 days (3-4 days if you are coming off a diet. This will be hard. This will stock up your fat cells, and both help you lose, and help to stave off hunger while on the VLCD (very low calorie diet).

Foods recommended to eat:

The idea is to load up on fatty items, more than carbs. You can eat carbs if you wish, but you really should concentrate on the fats more. Many people find this a bit confusing, and aren't sure what to eatHere are some sample foods to eat, both the 'healthy' fats and the 'unhealthy' ones. You choose which to eat, just make sure you eat a *lot* of them!!

- Healthy Cold Pressed Oils
- Drizzle Extra Virgin Olive Oil, Sesame Oil, Coconut Oil on everything!
- Avocados
- Nuts: Especially Walnuts, Macadamia Nuts, Pecans, Pine Nuts, in that order, can really boost your fat gram load
- Nut Butters & Tahini
- Seeds: Sesame, Sunflower, Pumpkin are all great!
- Peanut butter!!
- Coconut: The oil, the milk, the meat
- Olives: Green or black, and stuff them with Tahini!

- Eat foods that you crave that are especially high in fat such as Dairy Queen, cakes, cookies, custards, creams, pastries, chocolate, etc. as it has a psychological effect of saying good bye (for now!)
- cheeses, especially French cheeses that are creamy and fatty, like brie
- Bacon, eggs, sausage! Make huge omelets with meats and cheeses
- Pizza
- Chocolate
- Mexican food
- Focus on high caloric creamy foods.
- Drink whatever you want on your load days; including soda, beer, wine, liquor, sake, etc.

It seems exaggerated but it is very important to follow this to the letter as it will avoid future issues such starving during the low calorie phase.

Phase 2 or Very Low Calorie Diet

During this period, you must carry on taking your HCG dosage, and keep adjusting it if needed. You will be on a very low calorie diet around 500 calories a day.

The goal of this phase is to lose between 1 to 3 pounds a day while taking hCG hormones with either the injection protocol or the ingested serum protocol. During this time, there is a menu plan that is placed upon a person that consists of eating 500 calories total each day. By eating such a small amount of calories, the body is encouraged to break down stored fats, up to a pound and a half, and utilize those fats in producing energy for the body to run through the day. Now, here's the kicker for this phase: a person must be able to commit to this diet for 21 to 40 days, taking the hCG and following the diet

Remember to drink around 3 liters of water a day. It is recommended while this is going on to take potassium (99 mg 3 times per day) to help with sleep, hunger and to stave off cramps, as your body will shed potassium with all the water. You may also wish to consider taking magnesium as well to help keep you having regular movements (BM's). L-glutamine will help with cravings for 'comfort foods' too. If you have energy issues, consider B-12 to keep energy levels up.

Here you may follow the 3-week diet included in this book, which will keep you around 500 calorie a day. Alternatively you can also create your own diet, and as guidance here you have the calorie count for different foods:

Calorie count for different foods:

- Apple 15 cal/oz
- Orange 13 cal/oz
- Grapefruit 9 cal/oz
- Strawberries 9 cal/oz
- Asparagus 6 cal/oz
- Beet Greens 6 cal/oz
- Cabbage 7 cal/oz
- Celery 4 cal/oz
- Cucumber 3 cal/oz
- Lettuce, iceberg 4 cal/oz
- Onion, 12 cal/oz
- Radish 5 cal/oz
- Spinach 7 cal/oz
- Tomato 5 cal/oz
- Chicken Breast 31 cal/oz
- Flounder/Sole 26 cal/oz
- Halibut 31 cal/oz
- Scallops 25 cal/oz
- Shrimp 30 cal/oz
- Cod 23 cal/oz
- Ground Beef 95% 39 cal/oz
- Top Sirloin Steak 37 cal/oz
- Lemon Juice/wedge 1 cal/oz

Phase 3 or Maintenance Diet

When you have taken y our last HCG dose, write down you weight. Then stay for 72 hours longer on the very low calorie diet. Then the maintenance phase will begin, and your goal will be to stay within 2 pounds of the weight you wrote down after taking your last HCG dose.

No sugars or starches (which are carbs). You'll not be able to eliminate them, but you have to minimize them. This is critical to ensure a proper reset. Make sure you eat enough. A reason people cannot reset in this part of the protocol is by not eating enough. Keep drinking water. Water is essential to maintaining your weight and your health. Spend a couple days increasing to your recommended calories.

Now you must follow this:

- For 3 weeks following Phase 2, do not eat sugars or starches
- Eat to hunger
- Introduce calories/amounts of food gradually
- Introduce dairy, nuts, and fats slowly
- Keep your weight within 2 lbs of your VLCD
- If your weight goes above the 2lb window, start the three week Phase 3 period over again.

Phase 4 or Maintenance Diet

After 3 weeks of maintenance, you can start carefully adding in sugars and starches, remembering that you must stay within the 2lb limit above or below. Remember that you must reduce fats/protein when adding carbs, to keep in your calorie limits. Do this for 3 *more* weeks (minimum, and it lengthens depending on your round).

Your 3-Week Phase 2 Eating Schedule

Week 1

Week 1 Table Summary

	Monday	Tuesday	Wednesday	Thursday	Friday	Saturday	Sunday
Breakfast	*black coffee or tea—any size. + 1l. Water*	*1 cup strawberries and 8 oz green tea + 1l. Water*	*Instant oatmeal. Unsweetened, unflavored + 1l. Water*	*Cereals with blueberries + 1l. Water*	*Egg with mushrooms and bacon + 1l. Water*	*Fruit nut cereal + 1l. Water*	*Walnut oatmeal and yogurt + 1l. Water*
Snack	*Four grissine breadsticks* 8 oz Tea	*Carrots and salsa, cheese and an apple*	*Mango, cottage cheese and yogurt*	*Latte, banana, lemonade and popcorn*	*4 stalks of celery, Salsa, ½ apple*	*Yogurt, strawberries and olives*	Apricots and Ice-Cream
Lunch	Slow roasted beef brisket (100g)	*Turkey breast meatloaf*	*3.5 oz shrimp scampi and 5 melba toast rounds salsa*	*Turkey and avocado roll*	*Broccoli-cheese baked potato*	*Pesto turkey sandwich*	*Couscous Lentil Salad*
Dinner	Grilled Shrimp and Raab (100g)	*Chicken Cacciatore HCG (3.5oz) and 1 apple with stevia and cinnamon*	*3.5 oz Kund Pao Chicken. Salad greens. Fat free Italian dressing*	*Pork with pasta and green beans*	Chicken and Beetroot Salad	*Steak, sweet potato and veggies*	Grilled chicken and baked potato
HCG Treatment	*HCG Pellets/Pills After lunch*	*HCG Drops After breakfast*	*HCG Pellets/Pills After Dinner*	*HCG Pellets/Pills After Dinner*	*HCG Pellets/Pills After Dinner*	*HCG Drops After lunch*	*HCG Drops After Dinner*

Week 2

Week 2 Table Summary

	Monday	Tuesday	Wednesday	Thursday	Friday	Saturday	Sunday
Breakfast	*Apple + 1l. Water*	*Orange + 1l. Water*	*Apple + 1l. Water*	*Orange + 1l. Water*	*Apple + 1l. Water*	*Orange + 1l. Water*	*Apple + 1l. Water*
Snack	2 melba snacks	2 melba snacks	2 melba snacks	2 melba snacks	2 melba snacks	2 melba snacks	2 melba snacks
Lunch	Deviled Eggs	Mini meatballs	Garlic Lime chicken	Egg Salad	Curry Chicken	Garlic broccoli chicken stir fry	Scrambled eggs Florentine
Dinner	Stuffed Pepper	Taco Salad	Sloppy Joe	Chicken Spanish Tomato Soup	Beef Enchilada	Scrambled Eggs with Salsa	Chicken Fingers
HCG Treatment	*HCG Pellets/Pills After lunch*	*HCG Drops After breakfast*	*HCG Pellets/Pills After Dinner*	*HCG Pellets/Pills After Dinner*	*HCG Pellets/Pills After Dinner*	*HCG Drops After lunch*	*HCG Drops After Dinner*

WEEK 3

	Monday	Tuesday	Wednesday	Thursday	Friday	Saturday	Sunday
Breakfast	*Apple + 1l. Water*	*Orange + 1l. Water*	*Apple + 1l. Water*	*Orange + 1l. Water*	*Apple + 1l. Water*	*Orange + 1l. Water*	*Apple + 1l. Water*
Snack	2 melba snacks	2 melba snacks	2 melba snacks	2 melba snacks	2 melba snacks	2 melba snacks	2 melba snacks
Lunch	Fauxback Steak Rub	Garlic Lemon Chicken	Mini Meatloaf	Spaghetti and Meatballs	Chili	Cabbage Meatball Soup	Lemon Garlic Mahi-Mahi
Dinner	Chicken Spinach Tomato Soup	Garlic Lemon Chicken	Chicken Apple Slaw	Salsa Chicken	Sloppy Joe	Scrambled Eggs with Salsa	Scrambled Eggs with Tomato
HCG Treatment	*HCG Pellets/Pills After lunch*	*HCG Drops After breakfast*	*HCG Pellets/Pills After Dinner*	*HCG Pellets/Pills After Dinner*	*HCG Pellets/Pills After Dinner*	*HCG Drops After lunch*	*HCG Drops After Dinner*

Your 3-Week Phase 2 Eating Schedule

Week 1

Monday

Breakfast: Veggie Omelette made with 2 Whole Eggs, Shredded Cheese, Sautéed Tomatoes, Mushrooms and Onions and 2 pieces of Turkey Bacon

Snack: Apple with 1 TBSP Peanut Butter

Lunch: Large Salad with Chicken Breast and your choice of Salad Dressing, such as Ranch or Italian. (Remember all salad dressings used during the 1st 3 weeks of HCG Maintenance need to have 3 or less carbs, 2 or less sugars, and 12 or less fats)

Snack: Mixed Fruit Salad (avoid really sweet fruits like grapes, pineapple, etc.)

Dinner: Roasted Turkey (avoid Honey Baked or anything sweet) served with Steamed Green Beans and Mashed Cauliflower (substitution for Mashed Potatoes)

Snack: Fresh Strawberries dipped in Unsweetened Greek Yogurt

Tuesday

Breakfast: Cottage Cheese with Sliced Peaches (If canned, get all natural; NO added sugars) and 2 pieces of Turkey Sausage

Snack: Handful of Unsweetened Almonds (nuts are cautionary so start small)

Lunch: Cold Taco Pizza Recipe made with Flax

Snack: Sugar Free Yogurt (less than 10 grams of carbs), Plum

Dinner: Noodleless Spaghetti- Roast a Spaghetti Squash in the oven until tender. Combine with normal Spaghetti Meat Sauce. Top with grated Parmesan Cheese.

Snack: Carrots and Celery Sticks served with Ranch

Wednesday

Breakfast: 2 Eggs, Blueberries in Sugar Free Yogurt (less than 10 grams of carbs)

Snack: Mixed Nuts (nuts are cautionary so start small)

Lunch: Tuna Wrap- Prepare Tuna Salad as normal, then wrap in Lettuce. Served with a small Side Salad with dressing that is safe for the 1st 3 weeks of HCG Maintenance / HCG P3.

Snack: 2 Nectarines

Dinner: Stir-fry made with Shrimp, Broccoli, Bell Peppers, Onions, Carrots, Snow Peas, and Napa Cabbage sautéed in Soy Sauce

Snack: Apple with 1 TBSP Peanut Butter

Thursday

Breakfast: 2 Eggs Scrambled with Onions, Mushrooms, Pre-cooked Turkey Sausage, and Shredded Cheese

Snack: Unsweetened Greek Yogurt with Blueberries

Lunch: Bunless Burger- Burger Patty, Tomato, Pickles, Onion, Ketchup, and Mustard Wrapped up in Lettuce. Served with a small Side

Snack: Mixed Nuts (nuts are cautionary so start small)

Dinner: Two Meat Lasagna Recipe using Miracle Noodles

Snack: Unsweetened Applesauce with Cinnamon and Stevia

Friday

Breakfast: Almond Flour Pancake

Snack: Mixed Fruit Salad (avoid really sweet fruits like grapes, pineapple, etc.)

Lunch: Grilled Salmon, Steamed Broccoli and Edamame

Snack: 2 Hard-boiled Eggs

Dinner: Stuffed Peppers- Brown Ground Beef, add Sautéed Mushrooms, Onion and Peppers. Mix with Shredded Cheese. Put filling inside Bell Peppers. Cook in oven until tender.

Snack: Regular Flavored Pork Rinds

Saturday

Breakfast: Asparagus Frittata- Mix together raw Eggs (scrambled) with Chopped Asparagus. Pour into oven-safe dish. Top with Shredded Cheese. Bake until done.

Snack: Sugar Free Protein Shake

Lunch: Bunless BLT- Use the Lettuce to wrap together the Tomatoes and Bacon dress with 1 tablespoon Mayonnaise.

P3 Snack: Cottage Cheese mixed with Diced Tomatoes, Salt, and Pepper.

Dinner: Steak served with Steamed Carrots and Steamed Broccoli topped 1 tablespoon of Melted Cheese

Snack: Sweet Roasted Walnut

Sunday

Breakfast: Meat and Veggie Omelet made with 2 Whole Eggs, Brown Breakfast Sausage, Shredded Cheese, and Sautéed Tomatoes, Green Peppers and Onions.

Snack: Fresh Berries mixed with Unsweetened Greek Yogurt

Lunch: Soup made with Beef Broth, Stew Beef, Broccoli, Onion, Celery, Carrots and Seasonings

Snack: Sugar-Free Jello

Dinner: Butternut Squash Casserole Recipe

Snack: Celery with 1 TBSP Peanut Butter

WEEK 2

Monday

Breakfast: 2 Eggs, Banana

Snack: Mixed Nuts

Lunch: Lunch Wrap made with a Low-Carb Tortilla, Sandwich Meat, Lettuce, Tomato, your choice of Dressing

Snack: Cantaloupe Slices

DInner: Meatloaf, steamed Green Beans, and a small serving of Mashed Potatoes

Snack: Plain Greek Yogurt mixed with Strawberries

Tuesday

Breakfast: 1 cup of a Whole-wheat Cereal (Such as Kashi, Grapenuts, or Unsweetened Shredded Wheat) with ½ Cup Milk

Snack: Beef Jerky (Watch the Sugar Content)

Lunch: Cashew Chicken

Snack: Cheese Squares and Grapes

Dinner: Burritos- Ground Beef, Low-Carb Tortillas, Lettuce, Tomatoes, Onions, and Pico De' Gallo.

Snack: Low-Carb Protein Bar

Wednesday

Breakfast: Blueberry Nut Bread made with a Flour Substitute

Snack: Apple with Peanut Butter

Lunch: Tuna Salad, Served with Celery for dipping

Snack: Cottage Cheese with Berries

Dinner: Barbequed Chicken served with Low-Sugar BBQ Sauce, Corn, and a small Side Salad with your choice of Dressing

Snack: Pork Rinds dipped in melted Cheese Sauce

Thursday

Breakfast: Muffin Sandwich- 1 Whole-Wheat English Muffin toasted, with Deli Turkey Meat and Sliced Provolone Cheese. Warm in microwave until Cheese melts

Snack: Greek Yogurt mixed with your choice of Jam

Lunch: Zucchini Crust Pizza Crust topped with Tomato Sauce, Shredded Cheese, and your choice of Pizza Toppings

Snack: Trailmix (Mixed Nuts, Dried Cranberries, and Dried Cherries)

Dinner: Baked Chicken served with a Loaded Baked Potato (Topped with Melted Cheese, Bacon, Chives, and Sour Cream)

Snack: Applesauce with Cinnamon and Sweetener

Friday

Breakfast: Oatmeal or Kashi Cereal with Fresh Berries, Chopped Walnuts, and Sweetener

Snack: Celery with Peanut Butter

Lunch: Homemade Beef Vegetable Soup

Snack: Cottage Cheese with Grapes

Dinner: Un-sauced Chicken Wings served with Ranch or Bleu Cheese Dressing

Snack: Beef Jerky (Watch Sugar Content)

Saturday

Breakfast: Protein Shake, Orange

Snack: Deviled Eggs

Lunch: Chicken Fettuccini made with Miracle Noodles

Snack: Side Salad with your choice dressing

Dinner: Burgers on Whole-Wheat Buns served with Baked Sweet Potato Fries

Snack: Kiwi Fruit

Sunday

Breakfast: Ricotta and Strawberry Filled Flourless Crepes

Snack: Sugar-Free Jello with pears

Lunch: Sandwich on Whole-Wheat Bread with your choice of Deli Meat, Vegetables, and Low-Sugar Condiment (i.e. Mustard, Mayo, etc)

Snack: Chilled Shrimp and Cocktail Sauce

Dinner: Stir-fry made with Shrimp, Broccoli, Bell Peppers, Onions, Carrots, Snow Peas, and Napa Cabbage sautéed in Soy Sauce, served with White Rice

Snack: Greek Yogurt with Canned Mandarin Oranges

WEEK 3

Monday

Breakfast: Blueberry Nut Bread made with a Flour Substitute

Snack: Greek Yogurt mixed with your choice of Jam

Lunch: Meatloaf, steamed Green Beans, and a small serving of Mashed Potatoes

Dinner: Stir-fry made with Shrimp, Broccoli, Bell Peppers, Onions, Carrots, Snow Peas, and Napa Cabbage sautéed in Soy Sauce, served with White Rice

Snack: Applesauce with Cinnamon and Sweetener

Tuesday

Breakfast: 2 Eggs, Banana

Snack: Tuna Salad, Served with Celery for dipping

Lunch: Zucchini Crust Pizza Crust topped with Tomato Sauce, Shredded Cheese, and your choice of Pizza Toppings

Dinner: Two Meat Lasagna Recipe using Miracle Noodles

Snack: Sugar-Free Jello with pears

Wednesday

Breakfast: Oatmeal or Kashi Cereal with Fresh Berries, Chopped Walnuts, and Sweetener

Snack: Applesauce with Cinnamon and Sweetener

Lunch: Sugar Free Protein Shake

Snack: Carrots and Celery Sticks served with Ranch

Dinner: Burgers on Whole-Wheat Buns served with Baked Sweet Potato Fries

Snack: Side Salad with your choice dressing

Thursday

Breakfast: Protein Shake, Orange

Snack: Sugar Free Protein Shake

Lunch: Meatloaf, steamed Green Beans, and a small serving of Mashed Potatoes

Snack: Sugar-Free Jello with pears

Dinner: Noodleless Spaghetti- Roast a Spaghetti Squash in the oven until tender.

Snack: Tuna Salad, Served with Celery for dipping

Friday

Breakfast: Blueberry Nut Bread made with a Flour Substitute

Snack: Sugar-Free Jello with pears

Lunch: Cold Taco Pizza Recipe made with Flax

Dinner: Soup made with Beef Broth, Stew Beef, Broccoli, Onion, Celery, Carrots and Seasonings

Snack: Applesauce with Cinnamon and Sweetener

Saturday

Breakfast: 2 Eggs, Banana

Snack: Carrots and Celery Sticks served with Ranch

Lunch: Two Meat Lasagna Recipe using Miracle Noodles

Dinner: Burgers on Whole-Wheat Buns served with Baked Sweet Potato Fries

Snack: Applesauce with Cinnamon and Sweetener

Sunday

Breakfast: Oatmeal or Kashi Cereal with Fresh Berries, Chopped Walnuts, and Sweetener

Snack: Greek Yogurt mixed with your choice of Jam

Lunch: Zucchini Crust Pizza Crust topped with Tomato Sauce, Shredded Cheese, and your choice of Pizza Toppings

Snack: Sugar Free Protein Shake

Dinner: Meatloaf, steamed Green Beans, and a small serving of Mashed Potatoes

Snack: Side Salad with your choice dressing

THE RECIPES

Slow roasted beef brisket

Ingredients

- 2 tbsp sunflower oil
- 1.3kg (approximately) Asda Brisket Beef
- 2 large onions, cut into wedges
- 650ml beef stock made with 1 Knorr Rich Beef Stock Pot
- 2 tbsp tomato purée
- 2 level tsp mixed dried herbs
- 2 bay leaves
- 3 level tbsp gravy granules
- Roast potatoes, to serve
- Asda Smart Price Yorkshire Puddings, to serve
- Brocolli, to serve
- Carrots, to serve
- Peas, to serve

Preparation

1. Pre-heat the oven to 150C/130C Fan/Gas 2. Heat half the oil in a large pan and carefully brown the beef on all sides. Put in a large casserole dish.
2. Add the rest of the oil to the pan and cook the onions until soft and browned. Put in the dish around the beef.
3. Add the hot stock and tomato purée to the pan and heat until simmering. Pour over the meat and sprinkle on the herbs and bay leaves. Cover and cook in the oven for 4 hours, turning halfway through.
4. Remove the meat and vegetables with a slotted spoon and keep warm. Sprinkle the gravy granules into the juices in the casserole dish and stir to thicken.
5. Serve with the beef, roast potatoes, Yorkshire puddings, broccoli, carrots and peas.

Grilled Shrimp and Raab

Ingredients

- 1# Shrimp
- 2 bunches of Raab
- Sriracha

Preparation

1. Peel and devein 1# of shrimp
2. Preheat Grill
3. Blanche Raab in salted water and drain.
4. Lay Raab across the grill and season with salt and pepper, turning when they start to char. Repeat on the other side.
5. Season the shrimp and grill them.
6. Measure out 1 cup of Raab and 100g of shrimp serve with Sriracha.

Turkey breast meatloaf

Ingredients

Meat Loaf

- 1 1/4 lb ground turkey breast
- 1 container (6 oz) Greek Fat Free plain yogurt
- 1/4 cup ketchup
- 3/4 cup Progresso™ Italian style bread crumbs
- 1 tablespoon Worcestershire sauce
- 3/4 teaspoon salt
- 1/4 teaspoon ground sage
- 1/4 teaspoon pepper
- 2 cloves garlic, finely chopped, or 1/4 teaspoon garlic powder
- 1 small onion, chopped
- 1 egg, slightly beaten

Topping

- 1/2 cup ketchup
- 1/2 teaspoon ground mustard
- 1 tablespoon packed brown sugar

Preparation

1. Heat oven to 375°F. In large bowl, mix meat loaf ingredients. Spread mixture in ungreased 8x4- or 9x5-inch loaf pan, or shape into 9x5-inch loaf in ungreased 13x9-inch pan.
2. In small bowl, mix topping ingredients; spread over top.
3. Bake uncovered 1 hour to 1 hour 10 minutes or until meat thermometer inserted in center of loaf reads 170°F. Let stand 5 minutes; drain. Remove from pan.

Chicken Cacciatore HCG (3.5oz) and 1 apple with stevia and cinnamon

Ingredients

- 100gms chicken breast, diced (weight when cooked)
- 1 ½ cups tomatoes, chopped
- ¼ cup chicken broth or water
- 2 tablespoons tomato paste
- 1 tablespoon apple cider vinegar
- 2 tablespoons lemon juice
- 1 tablespoon Bragg's liquid aminos
- 2 tablespoons onion, chopped
- 2 cloves garlic, crushed and minced
- ¼ teaspoon onion powder
- ¼ teaspoon garlic powder
- 1 bay leaf
- Pinch of Cayenne to taste
- Stevia to taste

Preparation

Brown the chicken with garlic, onion and lemon juice in a small saucepan. Deglaze the pan with the chicken broth. Add tomatoes, tomato paste, vinegar, and spices. Simmer on low heat for 20 minutes, stirring occasionally. Remove the bay leaf and serve hot.

3.5 oz shrimp scampi

Ingredients

- ounces of Shrimp (peel shell off, weight out 3.5 ounces before cooking)
- 1/4 Tsp minced Garlic
- 3 Tbsp Fresh Squeezed Lemon Juice Dash of onion powder, garlic, salt and pepper to taste
- 1/4 Cup Vegetable Broth or Water (broth gives it more flavor)

Preparation

In saucepan sauté minced garlic in the lemon juice and vegetable broth. Add dry ingredients. Add shrimp and cook till pink or 5-7 minutes.

MELBA DELIGHT

Ingredients

- 1-2 Melba Toast/
- 4-5 Melba Snacks
- 1-2 Slices of chicken breast (deli style)
- 1 slice tomato
- Add oregano and a pinch of salt

Preparation

1 protein, 1 fruit/vegetable, 1 Melba
Roughly 75 Calories

Turkey and avocado roll

Ingredients

- 1/2pound sliced turkey
- 1/2cup basil pesto
- 1 avocado, thinly sliced
- 1/2package alfalfa sprouts
- 1teaspoon lemon juice
- salt and pepper to taste

Instructions

1. Sprinkle lemon juice, salt and pepper on top of the avocado.
2. Place one piece of turkey on cutting board. Spread with pesto, add avocado slice and alfalfa sprouts. Tightly roll up the turkey.
3. Slice each turkey roll in half, and serve.

3.5 oz Kung Pao Chicken

Ingredients

- oz (100g) raw chicken breast, cut into 1" cubes
- chopped onion (allowed amount)
- 3 cloves garlic, minced
- 1-2 tsp fresh ginger, minced or grated

Marinade (this is adaptable, I used 1/2 C each for 1 lb of chicken):

- 1 part soy sauce or liquid aminos (follow your plans recommendations)
- 1 part unseasoned rice vinegar

Other (these are the measurements I used for about 1/2 lb of chicken because I cooked the kids portions differently, see below):

- 1-2 Tbsp sambal oelek (chili paste)
- 1/2 C broth, plus more for cooking, if needed
- 1 Tbs soy sauce
- 1-2 tsp unseasoned rice vinegar

Preparation

1. In a dish appropriate for the amount of chicken you are using, mix the marinade ingredients and add the cubed chicken. Allow to marinate in the refrigerator for 30 min-1 hr.
2. Using a wok or other appropriately sized pan, stir-fry or saute chicken for about 5 min, browning all sides. If you don't use non-stick pans you made need to add small amounts of broth to keep the chicken from sticking or burning.
3. Add sambal oelek to pan and continue cooking for another 1-2 min.
4. Check chicken pieces to be certain they are cooked through, then remove to a bowl and set aside.
5. Add onion to pan and sauté until tender, again using broth if necessary. Add in garlic and ginger and cook for another 1-2 min. Add chicken broth, soy sauce and rice vinegar and continue to cook about 3 mins, allowing the sauce to reduce slightly. Put chicken back into sauce mixture and warm for 1-2 min more.

Pork with pasta and green beans

Ingredients

- 3 ounces uncooked angel hair pasta
- 1/2 pound boneless pork loin chops, cut into thin strips
- 1/4 teaspoon salt
- 1/4 teaspoon pepper
- 1 teaspoon canola oil, divided
- 1-1/2 cups cut fresh green beans
- 2 celery ribs, sliced
- 4-1/2 teaspoons chopped onion
- 3 tablespoons water
- 4 teaspoons reduced-sodium soy sauce
- 1 teaspoon butter

Preparation

1. Cook pasta according to package directions. Meanwhile, sprinkle pork with salt and pepper. In a large non-stick skillet or wok coated with cooking spray, stir-fry pork in 1/2 teaspoon oil until no longer pink. Remove and keep warm.
2. In the same pan, stir-fry the beans, celery and onion in remaining oil until crisp-tender. Add the water, soy sauce and reserved pork; heat through. Drain pasta; stir in butter until melted. Add pork mixture and toss to coat.

Broccoli-cheese baked potato

Ingredients

- 8 large baking potatoes
- 2 tablespoons olive oil
- 3/4 pound broccoli florets (5 cups)
- 1 large onion, finely chopped
- 4 cloves garlic, minced
- 2 cups grated low-fat Cheddar
- 1/2 cup sour cream
- 1/4 cup milk
- Salt and pepper

Preparation

1. Preheat oven to 375°F. Rub potatoes with 1 Tbsp. oil; pierce with a knife. Bake until tender, 1 hour and 30 minutes. Steam broccoli until tender, 5 minutes. Drain; rinse. Pat dry and roughly chop.
2. In a skillet over low heat, warm 1 Tbsp. oil. Sauté onion until soft, 10 minutes. Add garlic; cook 2 minutes. Remove from heat.
3. Let potatoes rest until cool enough to handle. Set oven to 350°F. Cut top 1/4 inch off potato. Scoop out flesh.
4. Mash potato flesh. Mix with remaining ingredients. Fill potato shells with mixture; bake 30 minutes.

Chicken and Beetroot Salad

Ingredients

- 250g thin-stemmed broccoli
- 2 tsp rapeseed oil
- 3 skinless chicken breasts
- 1 red onion, thinly sliced
- 100g bag watercress
- 2 raw beetroots (about 175g), peeled and julienned or grated
- 1 tsp nigella seeds

For the avocado pesto

- small pack basil
- 1 avocado
- ½ garlic cloves, crushed
- 25g walnut halves, crumbled
- 1 tbsp rapeseed oil
- juice and zest 1 lemon

Preparation

1. Bring a large pan of water to the boil, add the broccoli and cook for 2 mins. Drain, then refresh under cold water. Heat a griddle pan, toss the broccoli in 1⁄2 tsp of the rapeseed oil and griddle for 2-3 mins, turning, until a little charred. Set aside to cool. Brush the chicken with the remaining oil and season. Griddle for 3-4 mins each side or until cooked through. Leave to cool, then slice or shred into chunky pieces.
2. Next, make the pesto. Pick the leaves from the basil and set aside a handful to top the salad. Put the rest in the small bowl of a food processor. Scoop the flesh from the avocado and add to the food processor with the garlic, walnuts, oil, 1 tbsp lemon juice, 2-3 tbsp cold water and some seasoning. Blitz until smooth, then transfer to a small serving dish. Pour the remaining lemon juice over the sliced onions and leave for a few mins.
3. Pile the watercress onto a large platter. Toss through the broccoli and onion, along with the lemon juice they were soaked in. Top with the beetroot, but don't mix it in, and the chicken. Scatter over the reserved basil leaves, the lemon zest and nigella seeds, then serve with the avocado pesto.

Pesto turkey sandwich

Ingredients

- 1/4 cup fat-free mayonnaise
- 1 tablespoon commercial pesto
- 1 teaspoon fresh lemon juice
- 1/2 teaspoon dried oregano
- 1/8 teaspoon black pepper
- 4 (2-ounce) French bread rolls
- 2 cups trimmed arugula
- 8 ounces thinly sliced cooked turkey breast
- 8 (1/4-inch-thick) slices tomato
- 4 (1-ounce) slices part-skim mozzarella cheese

Preparation

1. Preheat broiler.
2. Combine first 5 ingredients.
3. Cut rolls in half horizontally; spread mayonnaise mixture evenly over cut sides of rolls. Divide arugula, turkey, and tomato slices evenly among bottom halves of rolls; top each with 1 cheese slice. Place bottom halves of rolls on a baking sheet. Broil 2 minutes or until cheese melts. Cover with top halves of rolls.

Steak, sweet potato and veggies

Ingredients

- 1 x 300 g beef eye fillet steak
- alioli, to serve

For the three veg

- 1 large potato, peeled and sliced with a vegetable peeler
- 1 sweet potatoes, peeled and sliced with a vegetable peeler
- 1 parsnip, peeled and sliced with a vegetable peeler
- 50 g butter, melted
- 40 g finely grated parmesan
- 1 tbsp thyme

Preparation

1. **For the three veg:** preheat the oven to 200C/180C fan/gas 6. Place the potato, sweet potato and parsnip in separate bowls. Divide the butter, parmesan, thyme, a pinch of salt and cracked black pepper among the bowls and toss to combine.
2. Line a baking tray with non-stick baking paper. Pile each vegetable into 2 flat piles. Bake for 20'25 minutes or until golden and crisp. While the vegetables are cooking, cook the beef.
3. **For the beef:** sprinkle the meat generously with salt and cracked black pepper. Heat a frying pan over high heat. Cook the beef for 3 minutes each side or until well browned. Place on a baking tray and bake for 4 minutes for rare and 7'8 minutes for medium. To serve, slice the beef in half and place on serving plates with the three veg. Serve with aïoli.

Grilled chicken and baked potato

Ingredients

For the roasted garlic-oregano vinaigrette:

- 8 cloves roasted garlic
- 1/4 cup white wine vinegar
- 2 tablespoons fresh oregano leaves
- 2 tablespoons fresh parsley leaves
- 1 tablespoon honey
- 1/2 teaspoon kosher salt
- 3/4 cup olive oil
- 1/4 teaspoon red chili flakes

For the grilled chicken and potatoes:

- 12 fingerling potatoes, scrubbed
- Kosher salt
- Olive oil
- 4 (8-ounce) bone-in chicken breasts
- Freshly ground black pepper
- Fresh oregano sprigs, for garnish
- Fresh parsley sprigs, for garnish

Preparation

For the roasted garlic-oregano vinaigrette:
Combine garlic, vinegar, oregano, parsley, honey and salt in a blender and blend until smooth. With the motor running, slowly add the oil and process until emulsified. Stir in the red chili flakes.
For the grilled chicken and potatoes:
Place potatoes in a medium saucepan, cover with cold water and add 1 tablespoon of salt. Bring to a boil over high heat and cook until a paring knife inserted comes out with some resistance. Do not cook the potatoes all the way through because they will continue cooking on the grill. Drain well and when cool enough to handle, slice in half lengthwise.

Heat the grill to medium.
Brush the chicken and potatoes with oil and season with salt and pepper. Place the chicken on the grill, skin-side down and grill until golden brown and slightly charred, 6 to 7 minutes. Turn the chicken over and continue grilling until just cooked through, 5 to 6 minutes. A few minutes before the chicken has finished cooking, place the potatoes on the grill, cut-side down and cook until lightly golden brown, about 2 minutes. Turn over and continue grilling about a minute longer. Remove the chicken and potatoes to a platter and immediately drizzle with the roasted garlic-oregano vinaigrette. Let rest 5 minutes before serving. Garnish with oregano sprigs and parsley sprigs.

Couscous Lentil Salad

Ingredients

- 1⁄2 cup red onion, chopped finely
- 1⁄4 cup lemon juice
- 2 tablespoons red wine vinegar
- 1 cup lentils
- 5 cups water
- 1⁄3 cup extra virgin olive oil, plus
- 1 tablespoon extra virgin olive oil
- 1 cup couscous
- 4 tablespoons fresh parsley, chopped
- 4 tablespoons of fresh mint, chopped
- 3 scallions, white and light green part only, sliced thin
- salt and pepper

Preparation

1. Combine red onion, lemon juice and vinegar in large bowl with a pinch of salt.
2. Put lentils and 4 cups of water in pot and bring to boil then simmer for 20 minutes or until lentils are soft.
3. Take off heat and let rest for 5 minutes.
4. Drain and add to onion mixture along with the 1/3 cup of olive oil.
5. Toss well.
6. Bring 1 cup of water to boil, add couscous, take off heat, cover and let stand for 5 minutes.
7. Fluff up the couscous by raking with a fork and adding slowly the 1 T of olive oil. Try to get rid of the clumps.
8. Add the couscous to the lentil mixture along with the parsley, mint and scallions.
9. Salt and pepper to taste.

Deviled Eggs

Ingredients

- 4 hardboiled eggs

Preparation

1. Slice 4 hardboiled eggs in half and remove the yolks. Discard 3 yolks. Mix 1 yolk with a small squirt of prepared mustard, pinch of salt and pepper, and a small splash of milk. Divide between 8 egg white halves and serve.
2. Rogue Alternatives: You can substitute Ranch Dressing for the milk, if you like. Sometimes I use two yolks instead of one, if I feel the need for extra protein.

Stuffed Pepper

Ingredients

- 3.5 oz Ground Beef
- 1 Tbsp Onion, minced
- 1-2 cloves Garlic, minced
- 1 Bell Pepper, top and seeds removed
- 1/4 cup Tomato Sauce
- 2 Tbsp Tomatoes, diced
- 1/2 tsp Basil
- 1/2 tsp Oregano
- salt and pepper to taste

Preparation

Preheat oven to 350*. Mix basil and oregano into tomato sauce and set aside. Cook ground beef with onion and garlic until done. Add diced tomatoes and stuff the pepper. Pour tomato sauce on top and bake about 25 minutes or until pepper is done as desired.

Mini meatballs

Ingredients

- 3.5 oz ground beef
- 1 Tbsp bread crumbs (this is the equivalent of your melba or grissini allowance. You can crush that if you prefer.
- 1 Tbsp milk
- 1/4 tsp onion powder
- 1/4 tsp basil
- 1/4 tsp oregano
- 1/4 tsp garlic salt
- pinch pepper

Preparation

Preheat oven to 425. Combine all ingredients in a bowl. Form into small balls (I get 8-10 in a batch.) Place on baking sheet and cook 7-9 minutes or until done. Drain on paper towels. I like to use a little P2 Ketchup for dipping.

Taco Salad

Ingredients

- 3.5 oz Ground Beef
- Spices of your choice, like cumin, chili powder, cilantro, etc.
- 2 cups Lettuce
- 1 Tbsp Ranch Dressing
- 2-3 Tbsp Salsa

Preparation

Brown ground beef. Add taco spices of your choice to taste. Mix ranch dressing with salsa. Serve over lettuce.

Garlic Lime chicken

Ingredients

- 3.5 oz Chicken Breast (I use 2 tenders)
- Garlic cloves, peeled (I used 10)
- 1 Tbsp Onion, chopped
- 1 Tbsp Lime Juice
- 1 Tbsp Water
- 1/2 tsp dried Cilantro (or a Tbsp of fresh)
- 1/2 tsp salty seasoning, I used Adobo (optional)

Preparation

Preheat oven to 350*. Place chicken in a foil-lined baking dish. Combine water, lime juice and seasonings and pour over chicken. Add garlic cloves and onion. Close foil and bake until chicken is done, about 25 minutes.

Sloppy Joe

Ingredients

- 3.5 ounces Ground Beef
- 1/4 - 1/2 cup Onion, chopped
- 1-2 cloves Garlic, minced
- 1/2 cup Tomato Sauce
- 1/2 tsp Mustard
- 1/2 tsp Oregano
- 1/2 tsp Basil

Preparation

Brown ground beef with onion and garlic until almost done. Add tomato sauce, mustard and spices, and simmer until thick.
Optional: Serve over broiled eggplant slices (about 1 inch thick).

Egg Salad

Ingredients

- 4 Hardboiled Eggs (discard 3 yolks), finely chopped
- 1 Tbsp Milk, Mayo or Ranch, depending on your comfort with bending the rules
- Squirt of Mustard
- Salt and Pepper to taste

Preparation

Mix everything up as desired and serve over lettuce leaves. Quick and yummy!

Chicken Spanish Tomato Soup

Ingredients

- 8 oz fat free Chicken Broth
- 2-4 cups Water (depending how thin you like your chicken broth)
- 15oz can Diced Tomatoes
- 2 cups fresh Baby Spinach, washed and chopped
- 1 portion cooked, chopped Chicken (I used 1/2 chicken breast)
- 1/2 tsp minced Garlic
- 1/2 tsp Basil
- 1/2 tsp Oregano
- Salt and Pepper to taste

Preparation

Combine all ingredients into saucepan over med-hi heat, adding spinach last; it only needs to simmer for 2-3 minutes.

The original recipe calls for mini-tortellini, which you can easily cook separately and add to the soup if desired (for the rest of the family not on protocol).

Curry Chicken

Ingredients

- 1/4 cup Chicken Broth
- 1/4-1/2 cup Water
- 1/2 cup Tomato Sauce
- 1-2 tsp Curry Powder
- 1/3 cup Onion, chopped
- 3.5 oz Chicken Breast, diced

Preparation

In a medium pot or pan, heat broth, water and tomato sauce. Stir in curry powder. Add onion and cook until chicken is done. Remove chicken and continue simmering broth until it reduces and thickens into a sauce. Pour over chicken.

Beef Enchilada

Ingredients

- 1 Tbsp Water
- 1 Tbsp Onion, minced
- 1 clove Garlic, minced
- 1/2 can Diced Tomatoes
- 1/2 tsp Basil
- 1/2 tsp Oregano
- 1/2 tsp Chili Powder
- 1 tsp Cumin

Preparation

3 ounces of beef (or chicken), cooked and shredded. See my previous note about preparing meat ahead of time.

Garlic broccoli chicken stir fry

Ingredients

- 3.5 oz Chicken Breast (I use 2 tenders)
- 10 cloves Garlic, peeled and smashed
- 1.5 cups Broccoli (I use fresh)
- 2 Tbsp Water
- 1 Tbsp Bragg's Liquid Aminos

Preparation

Steam broccoli for just about 2 minutes to slightly cook it. (Frozen broccoli may not need this step.) Stir fry chicken in water until about half done, add garlic and finish cooking chicken. Add broccoli and Bragg's, stirring to coat. Serve.

Scrambled Eggs with Salsa

Ingredients

- 4 Egg Whites and 1 Yolk, beaten
- 2-3 Tbsp Salsa

Preparation

Scramble eggs until almost done to your liking, and mix in salsa. Easy!

Scrambled eggs Florentine

Ingredients

- 4 Egg Whites and 1 Yolk, beaten
- 1/4 tsp Garlic Powder
- 1/4 tsp Onion Powder
- 1 cup Baby Spinach

Preparation

Mix all together. Heat pan and cook as you would scrambled eggs, until cooked as desired.

Chicken Fingers

Ingredients

- 3.5 oz Chicken Tenders (this is 2 tenders for me)
- 1 Tbsp Mustard
- 1/2 tsp Basil
- 1/2 tsp Oregano
- 1 Tbsp Bread Crumbs (you can crush up your melba toast or grissini, or just use whatever bread crumbs you have)

Preparation

Preheat oven to 350*. Coat thawed chicken in mustard and set on baking sheet. Mix bread crumbs with herbs. Sprinkle half of the breading over the two tenders, then flip them over and sprinkle the rest on the other sides. Bake until done, about 15 minutes.

Fauxback Steak Rub

Ingredients

- 4 tsp paprika
- 2 tsp black pepper
- 1 tsp cayenne pepper
- 4 tsp salt
- 1 tsp garlic powder
- 1 tsp onion powder
- 1/2 tsp turmeric
- 1/2 tsp coriander

Chicken Spinach Tomato Soup

Ingredients

- 8 oz fat free Chicken Broth
- 2-4 cups Water (depending how thin you like your chicken broth)
- 15oz can Diced Tomatoes
- 2 cups fresh Baby Spinach, washed and chopped
- 1 portion cooked, chopped Chicken (I used 1/2 chicken breast)
- 1/2 tsp minced Garlic
- 1/2 tsp Basil
- 1/2 tsp Oregano
- Salt and Pepper to taste

Preparation

1. Combine all ingredients into saucepan over med-hi heat, adding spinach last; it only needs to simmer for 2-3 minutes.
2. The original recipe calls for mini-tortellini, which you can easily cook separately and add to the soup if desired (for the rest of the family not on protocol).

Garlic Lemon Chicken

Ingredients

- Juice of 1/2 lemon
- 1 Tbsp onion, minced
- 1-2 cloves garlic, minced
- salt and pepper to taste
- Liquid Stevia to taste
- Bragg's Liquid Aminos to taste
- 3.5 oz chicken, cut up

Preparation

Heat pan, add lemon juice, onion and garlic. Cook for 1 minute. Add salt and pepper, a couple of drops of stevia and a squirt of Bragg's. Add chicken and stir to coat, then cook until chicken is done.

Mini Meatloaf

Ingredients

- 3.5 oz ground beef
- 1 Tbsp bread crumb
- 1/4 tsp garlic powder
- 1/4 tsp onion powder
- 1/4 tsp oregano
- 1/2 tsp basil
- 1/2 tsp prepared mustard
- 1 Tbsp P2 Ketchup with a couple of drops of liquid stevia mixed in
- Salt/pepper to taste

Preparation

Preheat oven to 350. Combine all ingredients and form into a small meatloaf. Place on small baking pan and bake 15-20 minutes or until almost done. Spread P2 Ketchup (I would add liquid stevia again) on top and bake 5 more minutes. Serve with additional ketchup for dipping.

Chicken Apple Slaw

Ingredients

- 1.5 cups Cabbage, shredded
- 3.5 oz Chicken, cooked and diced
- 1 Apple, diced
- 1 tsp Mustard
- 1 Tbsp Apple Cider Vinegar
- 5 drops Liquid Stevia

Preparation

Mix mustard, ACV and stevia in a container large enough to hold the other ingredients. Add cabbage, apple and chicken and toss to coat. Eat immediately or refrigerate for later.

Spaghetti and Meatballs

Ingredients

Spaghetti Sauce

- 1 Tbsp onion, minced
- 1-2 cloves garlic, minced
- 1/2 can diced tomatoes, or 1 fresh tomato, chopped
- 8 oz tomato sauce
- 1 tsp basil
- 1 tsp oregano
- Mix and simmer while you make your meatballs.

Meatballs

- 3.5 oz ground beef
- 1 Tbsp bread crumbs
- 1 tsp milk
- 1/4 tsp onion powder
- 1/4 tsp basil
- 1/4 tsp oregano
- 1/4 tsp garlic salt
- pinch pepper

Preparation

1. Preheat oven to 425. Combine all ingredients in a bowl. Form into small balls (I get 8-10 in a batch.) Place on baking sheet and cook 7-9 minutes or until done. Drain on paper towels and add to sauce.
2. You can add the noodles to the sauce pot to heat through, or if you prefer your zucchini to be crunchier, pour the hot sauce over the zucchini noodles.

Salsa Chicken

Ingredients

- 3.5 oz Chicken Breast (I use 2 tenders)
- 1/2 cup to 1 cup Salsa

Preparation

Preheat oven to 350*. Place chicken in baking dish, cover with salsa. Cover with foil and bake until chicken is done, about 20-25 minutes. Serve.

Cabbage Meatball Soup

Ingredients

- 1/2 cup Water
- 1/2 cup Fat Free Beef Broth
- 1 tsp oregano
- 1 tsp basil
- 1-2 Tbsp tomato sauce, optional
- 2 cups Cabbage, chopped or shredded

Mix water, broth and spices. Cook cabbage in broth until done.

Mix meatballs and bake while cabbage is cooking:

Meatballs

- 3.5 oz ground beef
- 1 Tbsp bread crumbs
- 1 tsp milk
- 1/4 tsp onion powder
- 1/4 tsp basil
- 1/4 tsp oregano
- 1/4 tsp garlic salt
- pinch pepper

Preparation

1. Preheat oven to 425. Combine all ingredients in a bowl. Form into small balls (I get 8-10 in a batch.) Place on baking sheet and cook 7-9 minutes or until done.
2. Drain meatballs on paper towel and add to soup. Super simple! Salt and pepper to taste.

Chili

Ingredients

- 3.5 oz ground beef
- 2 Tbsp minced onion
- 2 cloves garlic, minced
- 1 cup chopped tomatoes or 1/2 can diced tomatoes
- 1/2 cup water
- 1/4 tsp garlic powder
- 1/4 tsp onion powder
- 1/4 tsp chili powder
- 1/4 tsp cumin
- 1/4 tsp oregano
- Salt and pepper to taste

Preparation

Brown ground beef in small pan with onions and garlic. Drain fat if needed. Stir in tomatoes and water. Add spices, bring to a boil, then turn it down and simmer. If using fresh tomatoes, simmer until they cook down well.

Scrambled Eggs with Salsa

Ingredients

- 4 Egg Whites and 1 Yolk, beaten
- 2-3 Tbsp Salsa

Preparation

Scramble eggs until almost done to your liking, and mix in salsa. Easy!

Lemon Garlic Mahi-Mahi

Ingredients

- 1 Mahi -Mahi Fillet (mine come in 4oz portions)
- 3-4 cloves Garlic, smashed
- 1-2 Tbsp Lemon Juice
- 1 Tbsp Bragg's Liquid Aminos, optional

Preparation

Preheat oven to 350* (I use my toaster oven). Line a small baking dish with foil (you'll thank me later). Mix garlic in lemon juice (and Bragg's, if using) and pour over mahi. Bake about 20 minutes or until fish flakes easily with a fork. Serve!

Scrambled Eggs with Tomato

Ingredients

- 4 Egg Whites and 1 Yolk, beaten
- 1/4 cup Diced Tomato (I used canned)
- 1-2 cloves Garlic, minced
- 2 Tbsp Onion, minced
- Salt and Pepper to taste

Preparation

Cook tomato, garlic and onion together until the onion is done. Add eggs and scramble until cooked the way you like.

Made in the USA
Lexington, KY
04 July 2017